Male Infertility
Causes and Management

Akmal El-Mazny

Copyright © 2015 Akmal El-Mazny

All rights reserved.

CreateSpace, Charleston SC, USA

ISBN-13: 978-1505744729
ISBN-10: 1505744725

CONTENTS

INTRODUCTION	1
OVERVIEW	2
– BASIC ANATOMY	2
– BASIC PHYSIOLOGY	4
– GENERAL CONSIDERATIONS	12
CAUSES OF MALE INFERTILITY	15
– PRETESTICULAR CAUSES	15
– TESTICULAR CAUSES	20
– POSTTESTICULAR CAUSES	27
MALE INFERTILITY WORKUP	32
– HISTORY	33
– EXAMINATION	40
– INVESTIGATIONS	44
MALE INFERTILITY TREATMENT	54
– MEDICAL TREATMENT	54
– SURGICAL TREATMENT	59
– ASSISTED REPRODUCTION TECHNIQUES	67
– MALE FERTILITY PRESERVATION	71
REFERENCES	75

INTRODUCTION

Male factors are often the cause of a couple's failure to conceive, therefore, it is important to evaluate and treat the male partner.

A male factor may be due to abnormalities of hormonal control, testicular function, or sperm transport or delivery.

Evaluation of infertile men is essential to identify both correctable and uncorrectable conditions.

A thorough medical and reproductive history and physical examination are integral parts of the workup.

The semen analysis provides the basis for identifying the cause of male infertility, as well as planning additional testing and treatment.

Treatment options are based on the underlying etiology and range from optimizing semen production and transportation with medical therapy or surgical procedures to complex assisted reproduction techniques.

I hope this book will enhance your knowledge of male infertility, and you will be able to apply this information to your practice.

OVERVIEW

BASIC ANATOMY

The male reproductive system is a network of external and internal organs that has three major functions:

- Produce germ cells, called spermatozoa, for sexual reproduction,

- Deliver the male germ cells to the female reproductive tract; and

- Produce hormones that regulate reproductive function and secondary sex characteristics.

The testes are the primary male reproductive organ and are responsible for testosterone and sperm production.

Sperm produced in the testes is transported through the epididymis, ductus deferens, ejaculatory duct, and urethra.

The epididymis is where sperm mature, concentrate and are stored for five to six days in this segment of the tract.

The vas deferens is a secondary storage site for spermatozoa; its epithelium has important absorptive and secretory functions.

Accessory glands include the seminal vesicle, prostate gland and bulbourethral glands.

The seminal vesicle provides precursor proteins responsible for semen coagulation, supplies fructose to nourish the ejaculated sperm and secretes prostaglandins that stimulate motility.

The prostate gland secretes proteolytic enzymes to liquefy coagulum after ejaculation, alkaline fluid to neutralize acidic vaginal secretions and the high zinc content is antimicrobial.

The bulbourethral glands, also known as Cowper's glands, secrete mucus for lubrication.

The penis is made up of an attached root and a pendulous body.

The root consists of two crura attached to the pubic arch and the bulb attached to the perineal membrane.

The body consists of two corpora cavernosa and the corpus spongiosum.

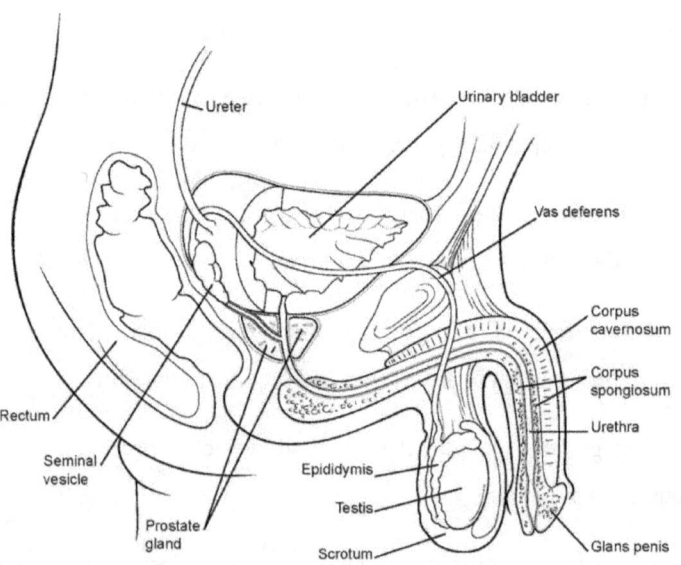

Male Reproductive System

BASIC PHYSIOLOGY

Hormonal Control

- GnRH is secreted by the hypothalamus and stimulates the pituitary to synthesize and release LH and FSH.

- LH stimulates Leydig cells to synthesize testosterone.

- FSH maintains Sertoli cell function.

Effects of Testosterone

Testosterone has significant reproductive and nonreproductive effects throughout the male life cycle.

Before birth, testosterone masculinizes the reproductive tract and external genitalia and promotes descent of the testes into the scrotum.

For sex-specific tissues, testosterone promotes growth and maturation of the reproductive system at puberty, is essential for spermatogenesis, and maintains the reproductive tract throughout adulthood.

Other reproductive effects include development of the sex drive at puberty and control of gonadotropin hormone secretion; secondary sex characteristics are also testosterone-dependent.

Testosterone induces the male pattern of hair growth (such as the beard), causes the voice to deepen due to thickening of the vocal cords, and promotes muscle growth responsible for the male body configuration.

Nonreproductive actions of testosterone include a protein anabolic effect, promotion of bone growth at puberty and closure of the epiphyseal plates.

Pituitary Feedback

Testosterone provides negative feedback to the pituitary to decrease LH and FSH levels, and to the hypothalamus to decrease GnRH production.

Testosterone only partially decreases FSH production; inhibin, produced by Sertoli cells, is responsible for the remainder of the inhibition of FSH production.

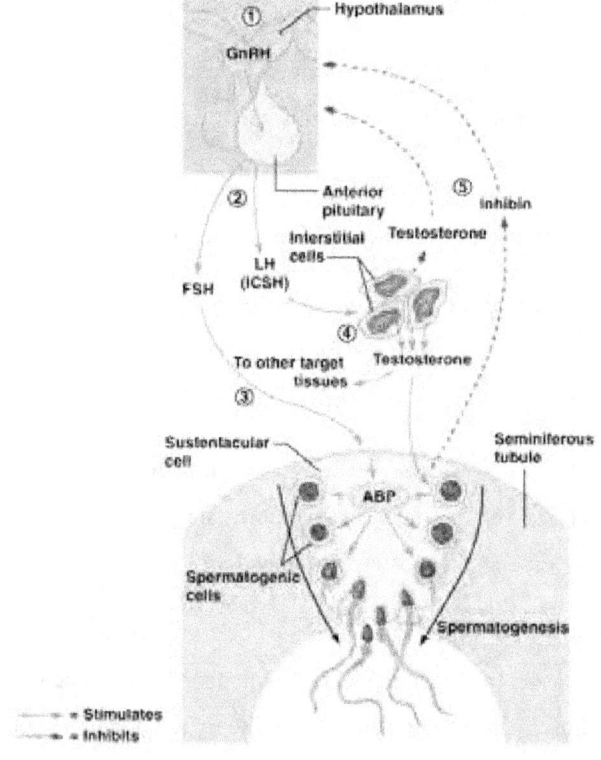

Hormonal Control of Testicular Function

Spermatogenesis

Beginning at puberty, spermatogenesis occurs continuously and repeatedly within folds of the Sertoli cells.

Spermatogonia lie at the base of the Sertoli cells and proliferate through mitosis to produce daughter cells that enter spermatogenesis.

In the two-step reduction division process of meiosis, spermatocytes and spermatids develop.

Spermatids are haploid, containing only one copy of each chromosome.

As the germ cells divide and mature, they move away from the base of the tubule toward the apical surface of Sertoli cells.

Spermatogenesis takes 74 days, with several hundred million sperm reaching maturity daily.

The process is temperature sensitive, occurring only at temperatures less than or equal to 36°C.

Spermiogenesis

Following meiosis, spermiogenesis is the maturation process in which the round spermatids are transformed into elongated spermatozoa with tails.

The spermatid nucleus condenses and most cytoplasm is lost.

The Golgi apparatus moves to one side of the nucleus, forming an acrosome that surrounds the top two thirds of the nucleus (in the head).

Cell microtubules organize into a flagellar apparatus to form the tail for motility, and mitochondria for movement.

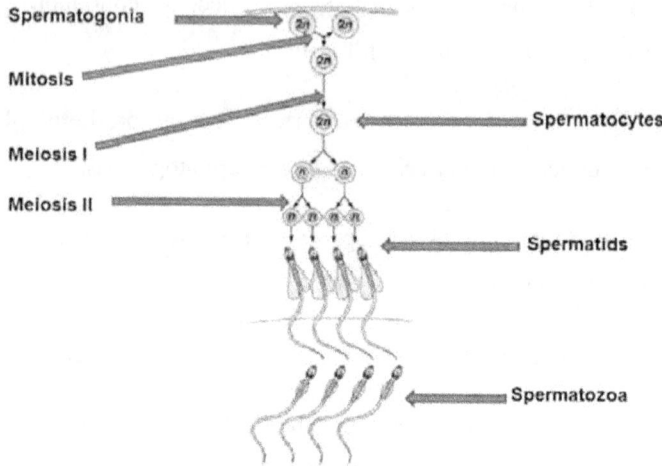

Spermatogenesis

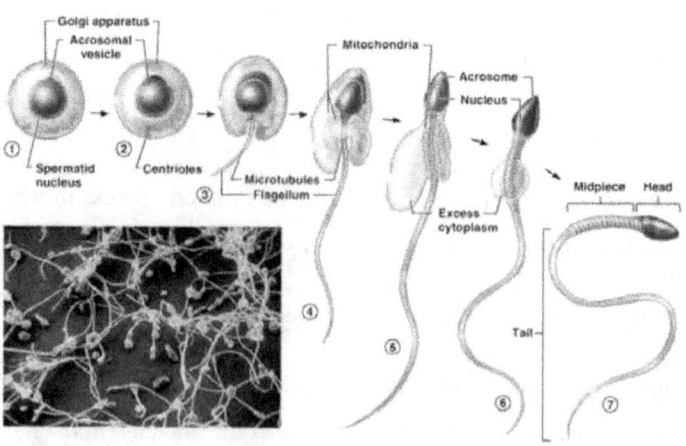

Spermiogenesis

Spermiation

Spermiation is the process in which fully developed but non-motile spermatozoa are released from the Sertoli cells and propelled out of the tubules into the collecting tubules, rete testis and then the epididymis.

Mature Sperm

Mature sperm have a head, which consists primarily of the nucleus containing genetic information.

The acrosome is a specialized lysosome, containing about 20 different enzymes, which are needed for penetration of the ovum during fertilization.

The acrosome covers the anterior third of the nucleus in a mature sperm cell.

In the midpiece are mitochondria to provide the energy required for the movement of the tail.

The tail grows out of one of the centrioles; movement results from the sliding of the microtubules.

Normal Sperm Morphology:

- The head is oval shaped, 4-5 microns long, 2-3 microns wide, the length-to-width ratio is 1.5 to 1.75, and a well-defined acrosome makes up 40 to 70% of the head area.

- The midpiece is intact and there is no cytoplasmic droplet.

- The tail is 45 microns long, and is not bent or coiled.

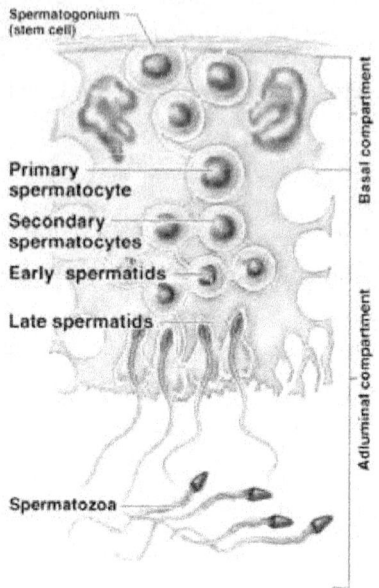

Spermiation

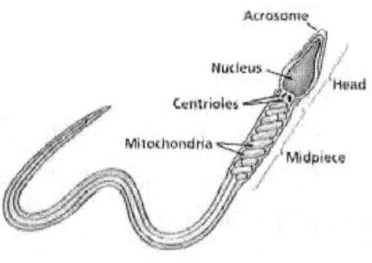

Mature Sperm

Erection and Ejaculation

The erectile bodies of the penis are composed of fibroelastic connective tissue, smooth muscle and a network of vascular sinuses lined with endothelium.

The sinuses are continuous with the arteries that supply them and the veins that drain them.

In the relaxed state, the central arteries in the cavernosa are constricted, limiting blood inflow; blood flows through sinusoids, and out through veins.

In the aroused state, the central arteries dilate and blood fills the sinusoids to compress the veins, reducing venous outflow and causing an erection.

Emission is a sympathetic and parasympathetic (S2-S4) event causing peristaltic waves up the vas deferens and contractions from the seminal vesicles and prostate gland to expel contents to the prostatic urethra.

Ejaculation is expulsion of the semen in the prostatic urethra distally down the urethra.

Ejaculation occurs by expulsion of the contents of the bulbourethral glands, followed by the fluid from the epididymis and prostate, accounting for about 30% of volume and the highest sperm concentration.

Lastly, the seminal vesicles empty and produce the largest portion of the seminal volume.

Semen is an admixture of sperm cells and secretions from the male accessory sex glands that combine at the time of ejaculation.

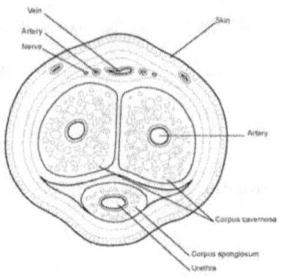

Cross-sectional Anatomy of Penis

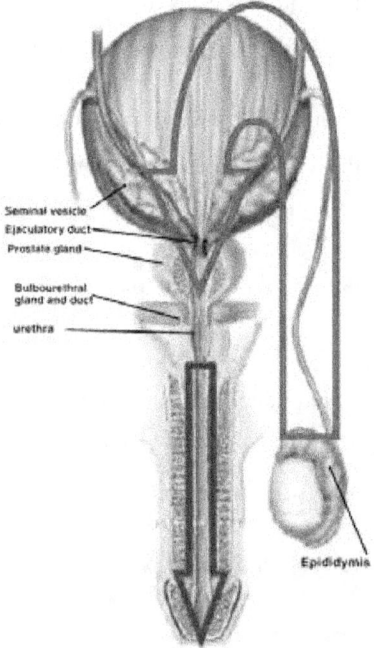

Mechanism of Ejaculation

GENERAL CONSIDERATIONS

Infertility is defined by the World Health Organization (WHO) as the absence of conception after at least 12 months of unprotected intercourse.

An estimated 10-15% of couples meets this criterion and are considered infertile.

Isolated conditions of the female are responsible for infertility in 35% of cases, isolated conditions of the male in 30%, conditions of both the male and female in 20%, and unexplained causes in 15%.

Conditions of the male that affect fertility are still generally underdiagnosed and undertreated.

Even if one partner has an obvious cause for the infertility, a thorough evaluation of both partners for completeness is prudent.

In addition, both partners may be aided by evaluation of their sexual practices.

Causes of infertility in men can be explained by deficiencies in sperm formation, concentration (eg, oligospermia [too few sperm], azoospermia [no sperm in the ejaculate]), or transportation.

This general division allows an appropriate workup of potential underlying causes of infertility and helps define a course of treatment.

The initial evaluation of the male patient should be rapid, noninvasive, and cost-effective, as nearly 70% of conditions that cause infertility in men can be diagnosed with history, physical examination, and hormonal and semen analysis alone.

♂ Infertility - *Overview*

History:

- Duration of infertility

- Previous fertility in the patient and the partner

- Timing of puberty (early, normal, or delayed)

- Childhood urologic disorders or surgical procedures

- Current or recent acute or chronic medical illnesses

- Sexual history

- Testicular cancer and its treatment

- Social history (eg, smoking and alcohol use)

- Medications

- Family history

- Respiratory disease

- Environmental or occupational exposure

- Spinal cord injury

Examination:

- Testicles (for presence, size, consistency, and bilateral symmetry)

- Epididymis (for presence bilaterally, as well as any induration, cystic changes, enlargement, or tenderness)

- Vas deferens (for presence bilaterally, as well as any defects, segmental dysplasia, induration, nodularity, or swelling)

- Spermatic cord (for varicocele)

- Penis (for anatomic abnormalities, strictures, or plaques)

- Rectum (for abnormalities of the prostate or seminal vesicles)

- Body habitus

Depending on the findings from the history, detailed examination of other body functions may also be warranted.

Semen Analysis:

The semen analysis is the cornerstone of the male infertility workup and includes assessment of the following:

−Ejaculate volume may range from 1.5 to 6.8 mL

−pH greater than 7.2

−Sperm concentration of 15 million/mL

−Total sperm number of 39 million per ejaculate

−Percent motility of 40%

−Normal morphology of 4%

More detailed, expensive, and invasive studies can then be ordered if necessary.

Treatment options are based on the underlying etiology and range from optimizing semen production and transportation with medical therapy or surgical procedures to complex assisted reproduction techniques.

CAUSES OF MALE INFERTILITY

Male infertility can be due to a variety of conditions, some of which can be identified and corrected, while others can be identified but not corrected.

When the male has an abnormal semen analysis for which the cause cannot be identified, the condition is termed idiopathic.

A male factor is almost always defined by abnormal semen parameters.

However, a male factor may also be involved when the semen analysis is normal.

A male factor may be due to hormonal abnormalities resulting in decreased sperm production, abnormalities of testicular function or abnormal sperm transport or delivery.

Causes of male infertility associated with normal sperm production include poor coital technique, erectile dysfunction, and ejaculatory disorders.

PRETESTICULAR CAUSES

Pretesticular causes of infertility include congenital or acquired diseases of the hypothalamus, pituitary, or peripheral organs that alter the hypothalamic-pituitary axis.

Disorders of the hypothalamus lead to hypogonadotropic hypogonadism.

If GnRH is not secreted, the pituitary does not release LH and FSH.

Ideally, patients respond to replacement with exogenous GnRH or HCG, an LH analogue, although this does not always occur.

Kallmann Syndrome

Some patients lack GnRH production and lack the nerves enabling their sense of smell, called anosmia.

Hypogonadotropic hypogonadism associated with anosmia is referred to as Kallmann syndrome.

Patients with GnRH deficiency do not produce LH and FSH, with resulting azoospermia.

Gonadotropin replacement therapy can reverse the azoospermia.

Abnormalities associated with Kallmann syndrome include anosmia, cryptorchidism, and gynecomastia.

Prader-Willi Syndrome

Prader-Willi Syndrome is a complex genetic condition that involves the loss of genes in a specific region of chromosome 15.

It results in low levels of FSH and LH, hypotonia, obesity, mental retardation, and short stature.

Laurence-Moon-Biedl Syndrome

Laurence-Moon-Biedl syndrome or Laurence-Moon syndrome is a rare inherited disorder characterized by diminished hormone production by the testes (hypogonadism).

Affected individuals have microphallus, hypospadias, undescended testes, and obesity.

Prolactinoma

A prolactin-secreting adenoma is the most common functional pituitary tumor.

Prolactin stimulates breast development and lactation; therefore, patients with infertility due to a prolactinoma may have gynecomastia and galactorrhea.

In addition, loss of peripheral visual fields bilaterally may be due to compression of the optic chiasm by the growing pituitary tumor.

A prolactin level of more than 150 mcg/L suggests a pituitary adenoma, while levels greater than 300 mcg/L are nearly diagnostic.

Patients should undergo an MRI or CT scan of the sella turcica for diagnostic purposes to determine whether a microprolactinoma or a macroprolactinoma is present.

Bromocriptine and cabergoline are dopamine agonists used to suppress prolactin levels.

These are both treatment options for microprolactinoma.

Some men respond with an increase in testosterone levels; many also recover normal sperm counts.

Transsphenoidal resection of a microprolactinoma is 80-90% successful, but as many as 17% recur.

Surgical therapy of a macroprolactinoma is rarely curative, although this should be considered in patients with visual-field defects or those who do not tolerate bromocriptine.

Isolated LH Deficiency

Isolated LH deficiency is also known as "fertile eunuch syndrome."

This is a variant of Kallmann syndrome where enough FSH is produced to induce spermatogenesis despite incomplete sexual development.

Isolated FSH Deficiency

This is a very rare cause of infertility.

Patients present with oligospermia but have LH levels within the reference range.

Treatment is with HMG or exogenous FSH.

Thalassemia

Patients with thalassemia have ineffective erythropoiesis and undergo multiple blood transfusions.

Excess iron from multiple transfusions may get deposited in the pituitary gland and the testis, causing parenchymal damage.

Treatment is with exogenous gonadotropins and iron-chelating therapy.

Cushing Disease

Increased cortisol levels cause a negative feedback on the hypothalamus, decreasing GnRH release.

Peripheral Organ

The hypothalamus-pituitary axis may be interrupted by hormonally active peripheral tumors or other exogenous factors, due to cortical excess, cortical deficiency, or estrogen excess.

Excess cortisol may be produced by adrenal hyperplasia, adenomas, carcinoma, or lung tumors.

High cortisol levels may also be seen with exogenous steroid use, such as that administered to patients with ulcerative colitis, asthma, arthritis, or organ transplant.

For example, high cortisol levels are seen in patients with Cushing syndrome, which causes negative feedback on the pituitary to decrease LH release.

Cortical deficiency may be seen in patients with adrenal failure due to infection, infarction, or congenital adrenal hyperplasia (CAH).

CAH may be due to the congenital deficiency of one of several adrenal enzymes, the most common of which is 21-hydroxylase deficiency.

Because cortisol is not secreted, a lack of feedback inhibition on the pituitary gland occurs, leading to ACTH hypersecretion.

This leads to increased androgen secretion from the adrenal gland, causing feedback inhibition of GnRH release from the hypothalamus.

Patients present with short stature, precocious puberty, small testis, and occasional bilateral testicular rests.

Screening tests include increased plasma 17-hydroxylase and urine 17-ketosteroids.

Estrogen excess may be seen in patients with Sertoli cell tumors, Leydig tumors, liver failure, or severe obesity.

Estrogen causes negative feedback on the pituitary gland, inhibiting LH and FSH release.

TESTICULAR CAUSES

Primary testicular problems may be chromosomal or nonchromosomal in nature.

While chromosomal failure is usually caused by abnormalities of the sex chromosomes, autosomal disorders are also observed.

Chromosomal Abnormalities

An estimated 6-13% of infertile men have chromosomal abnormalities (compared with 0.6% of the general population).

Patients with azoospermia or severe oligospermia are more likely to have a chromosomal abnormality (10-15%) than infertile men with sperm density within the reference range (1%).

Klinefelter Syndrome (47, XXY)

The most common sex chromosome disorder is Klinefelter syndrome, which is due to the presence of an extra X chromosome (47, XXY) and occurs in about 1 out of every 1000 males.

Men with Klinefelter syndrome have high FSH levels and may have low testosterone levels.

They characteristically have small, firm testes and azoospermia.

While some men have bilateral gynecomastia (breast enlargement), delayed puberty and a female body shape with relatively long legs, many men appear normal but only have small testes and infertility.

Some men have a mosaic pattern on karyotype (47, XXY/46, XY) and may have oligospermia.

XX Male

The 46, XX male is rare.

Although the karyotype is female, individuals are phenotypically males, with male external genitalia ranging from normal to ambiguous; two testicles; azoospermia; and absence of müllerian structures.

XYY Male

An XYY karyotype is observed in 0.1-0.4% of newborn males.

These patients are often tall and severely oligospermic or azoospermic.

This pattern has been linked with aggressive behavior.

Biopsy reveals maturation arrest or germ cell aplasia.

Noonan Syndrome

Noonan syndrome is sometimes referred to as male Turner syndrome and has autosomal dominant inheritance.

Defects in four genes (KRAS, PTPN11, RAF1, SOS1) affect proteins involved in the proper formation of several types of tissue during development, including sexual organs.

Individuals with Noonan syndrome typically have unusual facial characteristics, short stature, heart defects, bleeding problems, skeletal malformations and eye abnormalities.

Most with Noonan syndrome have normal intelligence, but puberty is usually delayed and most males have undescended testicles and diminished spermatogenesis.

Mixed Gonadal Dysgenesis (45, X/46, XY)

Patients have ambiguous genitalia, a testis on one side, and a streaked gonad on the other.

Y-chromosome Microdeletions

Y-chromosome microdeletions are found in 10 to 15% of men with azoospermia and severe oligospermia.

This condition involves the long arm (Yq11) of the Y chromosome.

There are 3 regions: Azoospermia Factor AZFa, AZFb, AZFc.

Deletion of the entire AZFa or AZFb region results in azoospermia.

Men with AZFc deletions may have azoospermia or oligospermia.

Bilateral Anorchia (Vanishing Testis Syndrome)

Patients have a normal male karyotype (46, XY) but are born without testis bilaterally.

The male phenotype proves that androgen was present in utero.

Potential causes are unknown, but it may be related to infection, vascular disease, or bilateral testicular torsion.

Patients may achieve normal virilization and adult phenotype by the administration of exogenous testosterone, but they are infertile.

Down Syndrome

These patients have mild testicular dysfunction with varying degrees of reduction in germ cell number.

LH and FSH levels are usually elevated.

Myotonic Muscular Dystrophy

Myotonic muscular dystrophy is an inherited disorder of progressive muscle degeneration.

It has an autosomal dominant pattern involving chromosome 19 and is the most common form of muscular dystrophy that begins in adulthood.

The condition causes hypergonadotropic hypogonadism, with elevated FSH and LH with low testosterone.

These men experience atrophy of the testicles and reduced fertility.

Congenital Deficiency of Testosterone Production

Congenital deficiency of testosterone production is a rare disorder that is caused by a lack of genes that encode for androgen enzymes biosynthesis.

There is incomplete virilization in affected men.

Nonchromosomal Testicular Failure

Testicular failure that is nonchromosomal in origin may be idiopathic or acquired by gonadotoxic drugs, radiation, orchitis, trauma, or torsion.

Varicocele

A varicocele is an abnormal dilation of the veins of the pampiniform plexus in the scrotum.

It is usually left-sided, but may be bilateral.

Varicocele is present in 15% of all males and in 40% of infertile males.

Varicoceles have a progressive deleterious effect on spermatogenesis.

This is the most common correctable cause of male infertility.

Cryptorchidism

In cryptorchidism, there is a failure of the testes to descend into the scrotum.

It is the most common birth defect of the male genitalia.

In boys born at full term, the cause is usually unknown.

About 30% of men with unilateral cryptorchidism and 50% of men with bilateral cryptorchidism will have oligospermia.

Androgen Insensitivity Syndrome (AIS)

Androgen insensitivity syndrome, or AIS, was formerly known as "testicular feminization."

In this condition, there is a defect in the androgen receptor gene, which results in a lack of androgen receptors, a defect in receptor function, or post-receptor defects.

Individuals with androgen insensitivity syndrome are genetic males (46, XY) but have a female phenotype.

Testes are undescended, there is a lack of pubic hair, and the proximal vagina, uterus and tubes are absent.

The condition affects 2 to 5 per 100,000 people who are genetically male.

Trauma

Testicular trauma is the second most common acquired cause of infertility.

The testes are at risk for both thermal and physical trauma because of their exposed position.

Sertoli-cell-only Syndrome

Developmental abnormalities include Sertoli-cell-only syndrome, also known as germ cell aplasia.

In this condition, there is congenital absence of germ cells in the seminiferous tubules of the testes due to failure of migration during embryonic development.

As a result, only Sertoli cells line the seminiferous tubules of the testes.

A pattern of Sertoli-cell-only can also be acquired as a result of exposure to chemotherapy or radiation therapy that destroys the germ cells.

Some men have small pockets of sperm production within portions of the testicle, which can be retrieved by testicular sperm extraction.

Chemotherapy

Chemotherapy is toxic to actively dividing cells.

In the testicle, germ cells (especially up to the preleptotene stage) are especially at risk.

The agents most often associated with infertility are the alkylating agents such as cyclophosphamide.

For example, treatment for Hodgkin disease has been estimated to lead to infertility in as many as 80-100% of patients.

Radiation Therapy

While Leydig cells are relatively radioresistant because of their low rate of cell division, the Sertoli and germ cells are extremely radiosensitive.

If stem cells remain viable after radiation therapy, patients may regain fertility within several years.

However, some have suggested that patients should avoid conception for 6 months to 2 years after completion of radiation therapy because of the possibility of chromosomal aberrations in their sperm caused by the mutagenic properties of radiation therapy.

Orchitis

The most common cause of acquired testicular failure in adults is viral orchitis, such as mumps virus, echovirus, or group B arbovirus.

Of adults with who are infected with mumps, 25% develop orchitis; two thirds of cases are unilateral, and one third are bilateral.

The virus may either directly damage the seminiferous tubules or indirectly cause ischemic damage as the intense swelling leads to compression against the tough tunica albuginea.

Normal fertility is observed in three fourths of patients with unilateral mumps orchitis and in one third of patients in bilateral orchitis.

Idiopathic Causes

Despite a thorough workup, nearly 25% of men have no discernible cause for their infertility.

POSTTESTICULAR CAUSES

Posttesticular causes of infertility include problems with sperm transportation through the ductal system, either congenital or acquired.

Genital duct obstruction is a potentially curable cause of infertility and is observed in 7% of infertile patients.

Additionally, the sperm may be unable to cross the cervical mucus or may have ultrastructural abnormalities.

Congenital Blockage of the Ductal System

An increased rate of duct obstruction is observed in children of mothers who were exposed to DES during pregnancy.

Segmental dysplasia is defined as a vas deferens with at least 2 distinct sites of vasal obstruction.

Congenital Bilateral Absence of the Vas Deferens (CBAVD)

In congenital bilateral absence of the vas deferens, or CBAVD, the vas deferens does not develop.

Many men with CBAVD also lack much of the epididymis.

This means sperm cannot pass from the testis into the ejaculate.

However, there is normal testicular function.

Congenital bilateral absence of the vas deferens is caused by a mutation in the CFTR (cystic fibrosis transmembrane conductance regulator) gene on chromosome 7.

CFTR functions as an ion channel across the cell membrane and is the same gene involved in cystic fibrosis.

All men with cystic fibrosis have CBAVD, and 80% of men with CBAVD have documented CFTR gene mutations.

Congenital bilateral absence of the vas deferens results in obstructive azoospermia, which is non-reconstructible.

Acquired Ductal Obstruction

Acquired ductal obstruction may be due to infections in the epididymis and ejaculatory ducts or from surgery, including vasectomy, radical prostatectomy, and transurethral resection of the prostate (TURP).

Antisperm Antibodies

The blood-testis barrier is a physical barrier between the blood vessels and the maturing sperm within the seminiferous tubules of the testes.

Connections between the Sertoli cells form a tight barrier that prevents passage of cytotoxic agents into the seminiferous tubules.

Disruption of this barrier by infection, surgery, or trauma can lead to anti-sperm antibody production.

Sperm-bound antibodies can alter sperm motility and decrease fertilization ability.

Genital injury can adversely affect sperm production or sperm transport and may also lead to anti-sperm antibody production.

Scrotal surgery can inadvertently lead to ductal obstruction.

Retroperitoneal surgery can injure the nerves responsible for seminal emission.

In testicular torsion, there is twisting of the spermatic cord, which cuts off the blood supply to the testicle.

As a result, sperm production may be impaired and anti-sperm antibodies may form.

Infections and sexually transmitted infections can result in tissue damage and ductal obstruction.

Common infections include orchitis (bacterial, or secondary to mumps), epididymitis (may be due to chlamydia or bacterial) and prostatitis.

Ejaculatory Duct Obstruction

Ejaculatory duct obstruction can be congenital or acquired.

Congenital duct obstruction is due to compression and obstruction of the ejaculatory ducts by cysts within the prostate, such as müllerian duct cysts or ejaculatory duct cysts.

Acquired obstruction may be due to infections such as prostatitis or epididymitis, or related to prior urethral surgery.

The obstruction can be partial, or complete with azoospermia.

Ejaculatory volume is low.

Ejaculatory Disorders

In retrograde ejaculation, semen enters the bladder instead of passing out through the urethra during ejaculation.

Anejaculation is the term for the inability, either physical or psychogenic, to ejaculate.

Causes of ejaculatory disorders include post-surgical changes, such as after prostate surgery or a retroperitoneal lymph node dissection (RPLND) performed to treat metastatic testicular cancer; neurological alterations, such as in diabetes; spinal cord injuries; and medications, such as alpha blockers for treatment of high blood pressure and some prostate conditions.

Psychological factors can cause premature ejaculation.

Erectile Dysfunction (ED)

Erectile dysfunction or ED, has become a well-known condition in recent years.

It is the inability to achieve or maintain an erection suitable for sexual intercourse.

ED can be a total inability to achieve erection, an inconsistent ability to do so, or a tendency to sustain only brief erections.

Erections begin with sensory or mental stimulation, or both.

Impulses from the brain and local nerves cause the muscles of the corpora cavernosa to relax, allowing blood to flow in and fill the spaces.

The blood creates pressure in the corpora cavernosa, making the penis expand.

As the tunica albuginea expands it compresses exiting veins to help trap blood in the corpora cavernosa, thereby sustaining the erection.

Development of an erection requires intact psychological, neurological and vascular mechanisms.

Physical causes of erectile dysfunction include cardiovascular disease, diabetes, neurologic disease, and hypogonadism.

Psychogenic causes include depression, anxiety, and stress.

Medications also affect ED, especially antidepressants and drugs to treat hypertension.

MALE INFERTILITY WORKUP

Goals of Evaluation

Identification and treatment of correctible conditions may improve a male's fertility and allow for conception via intercourse.

Evaluation will also identify uncorrectable conditions that may be treated with assisted reproductive technology using the male partner's sperm.

Detection of certain genetic causes of male infertility allows couples to be informed about the potential of transmitting genetic abnormalities that may affect the health of offspring.

It is also important to identify underlying medical conditions, such as testicular cancer and pituitary tumors, which can have serious consequences if not properly diagnosed and treated.

Timing of Evaluation

A male fertility evaluation should be performed when there is failure to achieve a successful pregnancy after 12 months of unprotected intercourse, or after 6 months based on history and physical findings or if the female partner is over age 35 years.

A fertility evaluation is also valuable for men concerned about future fertility, even in the absence of a current partner.

Initial Evaluation

The reproductive history should include the number of children, as well as a sexual and reproductive medical and surgical history.

Initially, at least one properly collected semen analysis should be performed.

Detailed Evaluation

Indications for a thorough evaluation include the following: an initial screening that reveals an abnormal history or abnormal semen parameters; couples with unexplained infertility; and couples who remain infertile after successful treatment of identified female factors.

Men should be referred to a specialist in male reproduction.

Components of a thorough evaluation for male infertility include a complete medical history, physical examination and additional tests if needed.

HISTORY

The initial step in the evaluation of an infertile male is to obtain a thorough medical and urologic history.

Important considerations include the duration of infertility, previous fertility in the patient and the partner, and prior evaluations.

The couple should be asked specifically about their sexual habits, including their level of knowledge of the optimal timing of intercourse and the use of potentially spermatocytic drugs and lubricants.

Patients should be asked about a history of childhood illnesses such as testicular torsion, postpubertal mumps, developmental delay, and precocious puberty, as well as urinary tract infections, sexually transmitted diseases, and bladder neck surgery.

A history of neurological diseases, diabetes, and pulmonary infections should be elicited.

Anosmia (lack of smell), galactorrhea, visual-field defects, and sudden loss of libido could be signs of a pituitary tumor.

The status of the partner's workup should also be known.

Timing of Puberty

Precocious puberty, defined as the onset of puberty before age 9 years in males, may be the sign of a serious underlying endocrinologic disorder.

Hormonally active tumors from the testicle, adrenal gland, or pituitary, along with adrenal hyperplasia, may result in early puberty.

In contrast, a delay in puberty may be caused by problems with testosterone secretion due to hypothalamic, pituitary, or testicular insufficiency or to end-organ androgen insensitivity.

Childhood Urological Disorders

Both unilateral and bilateral cryptorchidism are associated with a decrease in sperm production and semen quality, regardless of the timing of orchidopexy.

Patients with hypospadias may not place the semen at the cervical os.

Prenatal exposure to diethylstilbestrol (DES) may cause epididymal cysts and cryptorchidism.

Prior bladder neck procedure, such as a V-Y plasty performed at the time of ureteral reimplantation, may lead to retrograde ejaculation.

The vas deferens or the testicular blood supply may be injured or ligated at the time of inguinal surgery, hernia repair, hydrocelectomy, or varicocelectomy.

Testicular torsion and trauma may result in testicular atrophy and the production of antisperm antibodies.

Medical History

Diabetes may cause autonomic neuropathy, neurogenic impotence, and retrograde ejaculation.

Obesity alters hormonal metabolism, leading to increased peripheral conversion of testosterone to estrogen and decreased LH pulse amplitude.

Sickle cell disease may lead to sickling and, therefore, direct testicular ischemia and damage.

Patients with sickle cell disease or thalassemia may have infertility due to hemosiderosis from multiple blood transfusions.

Chronic renal failure leads to hypogonadism and feminization.

Liver disease may result in decreased male secondary sexual characteristics, testicular atrophy, and gynecomastia due to increased estrogen levels.

Hemochromatosis leads to hypogonadism and signs of androgen deficiency without gynecomastia and is associated with decreased estradiol levels.

Postpubertal mumps may lead to testicular atrophy.

Sexually transmitted diseases and tuberculosis can cause obstruction of the vas deferens or epididymis.

Mycoplasma fastens itself to sperm, decreasing sperm motility.

Smallpox, prostatitis, orchitis, seminal vesiculitis, and urethritis may lead to obstructive azoospermia.

Acute and Chronic Illnesses

Patients should be asked about recent acute febrile illnesses, which may temporarily suppress gonadotropin release.

Anesthesia, surgery, starvation, myocardial infarction, hepatic coma, head injury, stroke, respiratory failure, congestive heart failure, sepsis, and burns are associated with a suppression of gonadotropin release, possibly through an increase in dopamine and opiate levels.

Chronic medical illnesses may directly suppress sex hormone production and sperm production, leading to end-organ failure.

Respiratory Disease

Infertility and recurrent respiratory infections may be due to immotile cilia syndrome, which may be isolated or part of Kartagener syndrome (with situs inversus).

CF is associated with congenital bilateral absence of the vas deferens (CBAVD), leading to obstructive azoospermia.

While both copies of this recessive gene are necessary for clinical disease, the presence of only one copy may lead to CBAVD.

Young syndrome results in recurrent pulmonary infections and azoospermia due to inspissated material in the epididymis causing obstruction.

Medicines

Spironolactone, cyproterone, ketoconazole, and cimetidine have antiandrogenic properties.

Tetracycline lowers testosterone levels 20%.

Nitrofurantoin depresses spermatogenesis.

Sulfasalazine leads to a reversible decrease in sperm motility and density.

Colchicine, methadone, methotrexate, phenytoin, thioridazine, and calcium channel blockers have all be associated with infertility.

Testicular Cancer

Testicular cancer is associated with impaired spermatogenic function, even before orchiectomy, with a degree of dysfunction higher than that explained by local tumor effect.

Oligospermia is observed in more than 60% of patients at the time of diagnosis of testicular cancer.

Germ cell tumors may to share common etiological factors with testicular dysfunction, such as testicular dysgenesis, androgen insensitivity, and cryptorchidism.

Contralateral abnormalities of spermatogenesis are more common in patients with testicular cancer.

Sperm function often remains impaired, even after orchiectomy.

Retroperitoneal lymph node dissection (RPLND) may impair emission (of semen into the urethra) and/or cause retrograde ejaculation.

Chemotherapy, such as cyclophosphamide, mustine, and chlorambucil, severely alter the seminiferous tubules and destroy spermatogonia.

Radiation therapy may cause irreversible spermatocytes damage, although complete recovery may be possible if stem cell numbers are not depleted.

Spinal Cord Injury

Severe spinal cord injury may lead to anejaculation.

Epididymal and testicular factors appear to play a role, although the most severe dysfunction seems to come from prostatic and seminal vesicle dysfunction.

In addition, the semen quality in patients with a spinal cord injury may gradually decline owing to unknown causes.

This is hypothesized to be due to accessory gland dysfunction rather than lack of ejaculation and atrophy.

Sexual History

The frequency, timing, and methods of coitus and knowledge of the ovulatory cycle should be elicited.

Studies show that the optimal timing for intercourse is every 48 hours at mid cycle.

Lubricants such as KY Jelly are spermatotoxic, whereas egg whites, peanut oil, vegetable oil, and petroleum jelly are not known to be spermatotoxic but still should be used in only the smallest amounts possible if needed for lubrication during intercourse.

Family History

Congenital midline defects, cryptorchidism, hypogonadotropism, and testicular atrophy in family members may be a sign of a congenital disease.

A history of CF or hypogonadism should be elicited.

Social History

Cigarette and marijuana smoking lead to a decrease in sperm density, motility, and morphology.

Alcohol produces both an acute and a chronic decrease in testosterone secretion.

Emotional stress blunts GnRH release, leading to hypogonadism.

Excessive heat exposure from saunas, hot tubs, or the work environment may cause a temporary decrease in sperm production.

Contrary to widely held beliefs, no evidence supports that wearing constrictive underwear decreases fertility, even with an elevation in temperature of 0.8-1°

Environmental and/or Occupational Exposure

Many pesticides have estrogen-like effects.

Dibromochloropropane (DBCP) is a nematocide widely used in agriculture that causes azoospermia without recovery by an unknown mechanism.

Lead exposure depresses the hypothalamic-pituitary axis.

Carbon disulfide exposure from the rayon industry leads to semen, pituitary, and hypothalamic changes.

Heat exposure, as seen in workers in the steel and ceramic fields, decreases spermatocyte maturation.

EXAMINATION

The physical examination should include a thorough inspection of the testicles, penis, secondary sexual characteristics, and body habitus.

It should include a detailed examination of other body functions based on the history.

Testicles

The testicular examination should occur in a warm room with the patient relaxed.

The testicles should be palpated individually between the thumb and first 2 fingers.

The examiner should note the presence, size, and consistency of the testicles, and the testicles should be compared with each other.

A Prader orchidometer or ultrasonography may be used to estimate the testicular volume, with normal considered to be greater than 20 mL.

Calipers may be used to measure testicular length, which is usually greater than 4 cm, although the lower limits of normal length (mean minus 2 standard deviations) is 31 mm in white men and 34 mm in black men.

The testes of Japanese men are typically smaller than the testes of white men.

Testicular atrophy may be observed in primary testicular failure, Klinefelter syndrome, endocrinopathies, postpubertal mumps, liver disease, and myotonic dystrophy.

Swelling with pain indicates orchitis, whereas nontender enlargement may be observed in testicular neoplasms, tuberculosis, and tertiary syphilis.

Epididymis

The head, body, and tail of the epididymis should be palpated and assessed for their presence bilaterally.

Note induration and cystic changes.

An enlarged indurated epididymis with a cystic component should alert the examiner to the possibility of ductal obstruction.

Tenderness may be due to epididymitis.

Vas Deferens

Evaluate the vas for its presence bilaterally and palpate along its entire length to check for defects, segmental dysplasia, induration, nodularity, or swelling.

The complete absence bilaterally is observed almost exclusively in patients with either one or two copies of the gene for CF, although even a small defect or gap indicates the possibility of a CF gene mutation.

A thickened nodular vas deferens may be observed in patients with a history of tuberculosis.

If a prior vasectomy has been performed, the presence of a nodular sperm granuloma at the proximal vasal end should be assessed.

Spermatic Cord

Check patients for the presence of a varicocele, which is the most common surgically correctable cause of infertility.

To elicit this, the patient should perform a Valsalva maneuver in the sitting and standing positions in a warm room.

Grade 1 varicocele is defined as palpable only with Valsalva, while grade 2 is palpable at standing, and grade 3 is visible at rest.

The presence of asymmetry or an impulse with Valsalva may best help the examiner find a varicocele.

The sudden onset of a varicocele, a solitary right-sided varicocele, or a varicocele that does not change with Valsalva indicates the possibility of a retroperitoneal neoplastic process or vein thrombosis.

Penis

The examination should focus on the location and patency of the urethral meatus and the presence of meatal strictures.

Patients with hypospadias or epispadias may not deposit semen appropriately at the cervix.

Penile curvature and the presence of penile plaques should be noted.

Body Habitus

A eunuchoid body habitus, consisting of infantile hair distribution, poor muscle development, and a long lower body due to a delayed closure of the epiphyseal plates, may be observed in patients with endocrinological disorders.

Truncal obesity, striae, and moon facies may be due to Cushing syndrome.

Gynecomastia, galactorrhea, headaches, and a loss of visual fields may be observed in patients with pituitary adenomas.

Focus the neck examination on thyromegaly and bruits.

Palpate the liver for hepatomegaly.

Examine the lymph nodes to rule out lymphoma.

Rectal Examination

The prostate should be of normal size and without cysts, induration, or masses.

The seminal vesicles are usually not palpable.

A midline prostatic cyst or palpable seminal vesicles may be due to obstruction of the ejaculatory ducts.

INVESTIGATIONS

Laboratory Investigations

Semen Analysis

The semen analysis is the cornerstone of the laboratory evaluation of the infertile male.

Common instructions for semen collection are: 2 to 5 days of abstinence, with masturbation or intercourse using a special collection container / condom.

If the specimen is collected at home, it should be kept at room or body temperature and analyzed within 1 hour.

The semen analysis provides information on semen volume, concentration, motility and morphology.

Methods for semen analysis and laboratory protocols are defined by the World Health Organization (WHO).

The diagnosis of azoospermia is made only after centrifugation and examination of the pellet.

Reference values for semen parameters are not the same as the minimum values required for conception.

Men with semen parameters outside the reference ranges may be fertile and, conversely, men with values in range may be infertile.

In general, the more semen parameters that are abnormal, the more likely it is that a man will be infertile.

The following are the WHO 2010 lower reference values for semen analyses:

– Ejaculate volume may range from 1.5 to 6.8 mL

– pH greater than 7.2

– Sperm concentration of 15 million/mL

– Total sperm number of 39 million per ejaculate

– Percent motility of 40%

– Normal morphology of 4%

Abnormalities of semen analyses:

– Aspermia = no semen is present

– Azoospermia = semen is present but there are no sperm in the semen

– Severe oligospermia = less than 5 million sperm/mL

– Asthenospermia = reduced sperm motility

– Teratospermia = abnormal sperm morphology

Post-ejaculatory Urinalysis

A post-ejaculatory urinalysis is indicated for men with low-volume or absent ejaculate.

This may be due to retrograde ejaculation, lack of emission, ejaculatory duct obstruction, hypogonadism, or congenital absence of the vas deferens (CBAVD).

A post-ejaculatory urinalysis should be performed in men with ejaculation volumes of less than 1 mL, normal hormone levels and normal vasa.

For a post-ejaculatory urinalysis, urine should be collected after ejaculation.

The specimen is centrifuged for 10 minutes, preferably at 3000 g., and the pellet is examined at 400x magnification.

In men with azoospermia or aspermia, any sperm in the urine suggests retrograde ejaculation.

Quantitation of White Blood Cells in Semen

Increased number of white blood cells in semen is associated with poor sperm function and motility.

Under wet-mount microscopy, immature germ cells and leukocytes appear the same and are called "round cells."

The use of cytologic and immunohistochemical staining helps distinguish between the two.

Men with pyospermia (greater than 1 million leukocytes/mL) should be evaluated for genital tract infection or inflammation.

Sperm Viability Tests

Sperm viability tests are indicated when the sperm motility is less than 5%.

These tests help determine whether non-motile sperm are viable.

Eosin Y and trypan blue dye tests identify intact cell membranes in viable sperm by the ability of the cell to exclude the stain and remain colorless.

Sperm used in this test cannot be used in IVF.

In the hypoosmotic swelling test (HOS), viable sperm with intact cell-membrane function swell when placed in a hypoosmotic solution.

Sperm from this test can be used for IVF.

Sperm DNA Fragmentation Tests

Sperm DNA fragmentation tests help determine DNA integrity, which is important for embryo development.

DNA fragmentation refers to double-stranded breaks in sperm DNA that cannot be repaired.

Sperm DNA damage is more common in infertile men and may contribute to poor reproduction in some couples.

DNA fragmentation rates can be measured by either direct or indirect testing.

At this time there is no proven role for routine use of this test in the evaluation of male infertility.

Antisperm Antibodies (ASA) Testing

ASA testing should be performed if there is isolated asthenospermia with normal sperm concentration or sperm agglutination.

ASA can be found in serum, seminal plasma, or directly bound to sperm.

These antibodies form when there is breakdown of the blood-testis barrier due to trauma, infection, surgery or testicular cancer.

Detection of sperm-bound antisperm antibodies is made by a direct immunobead-binding test.

The antisperm antibodies bound to sperm head or tail are clinically the most important.

Endocrine Evaluation

The male endocrine evaluation tests the hypothalamic-pituitary-testicular axis.

As endocrine disorders are uncommon in men with normal semen parameters, testing is indicated in men with abnormal semen parameters (sperm concentrations <10 million/mL), impaired sexual function, and clinical findings that suggest specific endocrinopathy.

The minimum initial endocrine evaluation should include serum FSH and total testosterone levels.

If the total testosterone level is low (<300 ng/mL), LH, prolactin levels and morning bioavailable testosterone levels should be obtained.

Reproductive endocrine levels may vary depending on the clinical condition.

In hypogonadotropic hypogonadism, all levels will be low except for prolactin.

Elevated FSH levels are associated with decreased spermatogenesis.

In testicular failure, FSH and LH are elevated (hypergonadotropic hypogonadism).

With a prolactin-secreting pituitary tumor, testosterone, LH, and FSH levels are low, and prolactin levels are elevated.

Genetic Screening

Genetic abnormalities may cause infertility by affecting sperm production or sperm transport.

Men with nonobstructive azoospermia and severe oligospermia (<5 million/mL) are at a higher risk than fertile men for having a genetic abnormality.

The most common genetic abnormalities that cause decreased sperm production are numeric and structural chromosomal aberrations and Y-chromosome microdeletions.

Men with obstructive azoospermia due to congenital bilateral absence of the vas deferens (CBAVD) most commonly have an abnormality of the cystic fibrosis transmembrane conductance regulator gene (CFTR).

Identifying the underlying genetic cause of infertility can play a significant role in determining treatment.

Cystic Fibrosis Gene Mutation

There is a strong association between CBAVD and CFTR gene mutations.

All men with CBAVD are assumed to have a CFTR gene mutation.

The female partner must be genetically tested to determine the risk of conceiving a child with cystic fibrosis.

Prevalence of CFTR mutations is also higher in men with azoospermia due to congenital bilateral epididymal obstruction and those with unilateral vasal agenesis.

Karyotypic Chromosome Abnormalities

Karyotypic chromosome abnormalities are identified in approximately 7% of infertile men.

The frequency increases in proportion to the sperm count.

Abnormalities are seen in less than 1% of men with normal sperm concentration, 5% of oligospermic men and in 10-15% of azoospermic men.

Sex chromosome aneuploidy (Klinefelter syndrome 47, XXY) accounts for two-thirds of the chromosomal anomalies seen in infertile men.

The prevalence of structural abnormalities of the autosomes (inversions, translocations) is also higher in infertile men.

Men with severe oligospermia or nonobstructive azoospermia should have karyotypes before IVF with intracytoplasmic sperm injection (ICSI) using their sperm.

Y-chromosome Microdeletions

Microdeletions of sections of the Y-chromosome can be found in 10-15% of men with azoospermia or severe oligospermia.

These occur in regions of the long arm of the Y-chromosome (Yq11), known as the azoospermia factor (AZF) regions, which contain genes necessary for spermatogenesis: AZFa is the proximal region, AZFb is the central region, and AZFc is the distal region of the arm.

The DAZ (deleted in azoospermia) gene is in the AZFc region.

Men with AZFc deletions may have severe oligospermia, or azoospermia with enough testicular sperm for retrieval.

Men with AZFa or AZFb deletions have azoospermia, and a poor prognosis for testicular sperm retrieval.

Sons of men with Y-chromosome microdeletions will inherit the abnormality and may be infertile.

Y-chromosome analysis should be offered to men with nonobstructive azoospermia and severe oligospermia before ICSI using their sperm.

Imaging Studies

Ultrasonography

Transrectal ultrasound is used to evaluate seminal vesicle diameter, ejaculatory duct dilation, and to assess the prostate for cysts.

It can help diagnose ejaculatory duct obstruction and may be used in men with low volume azoospermic ejaculates, palpable vasa and normal testicular size.

Scrotal ultrasound is used to identify varicoceles and epididymal dilation, and can identify testicular tumors.

Color-flow ultrasonography is used to evaluate for varicocele using a 7- to 10-MHz probe.

A varicocele is diagnosed on a sonogram if a spermatic vein is greater than 3 mm or vein size increases with Valsalva.

Vasography

Vasography is used to evaluate patency of the ductal system.

Indications for vasography include azoospermia with mature spermatids present on testicular biopsy and at least one palpable vas.

Relative indications include severe oligospermia with a normal finding on testis biopsy, antisperm antibodies, and decreased semen viscosity.

This test may be performed either as an open procedure at the same time as testicular biopsy or by a percutaneous puncture.

Unilateral patency rules out vasal or ejaculatory duct obstruction as the cause of azoospermia.

Testicular Biopsy and Histology

Testicular biopsy is indicated in azoospermic men with a normal-sized testis and normal hormonal studies to evaluate for ductal obstruction, to further evaluate idiopathic infertility, and to retrieve sperm.

Primary testicular failure causes various defects.

Normal-sized seminiferous tubules, normal Leydig cells and Sertoli cells, and a normal tunica propria characterize maturation arrest, but germ cells are arrested at any premature stage.

Patients with hypospermatogenesis have a thin germinal epithelium and a decreased number of germinal elements.

Germ cell aplasia (Sertoli-cell-only syndrome) is associated with vacuolated Sertoli cells and no germinal epithelium but otherwise normal seminiferous tubules.

Klinefelter syndrome is characterized by a decreased number of spermatogonia, germ cell hypoplasia, Sertoli cell atrophy, tubular hyalinization, prominent Leydig cells (hyperplasia), and deformed tubules.

Cryptorchid testes have small immature tubules, spermatogonia of variable size, and a hyalinized tunica propria.

Acute mumps orchitis is associated with interstitial edema, mononuclear infiltrate, and a degeneration of germinal epithelium, while recovery is characterized by a patchy loss of germ cells with tubular hyalinization and sclerosis.

Biopsy samples in patients with infertility due to pretesticular causes have atrophic cells due to a lack of gonadotropin stimuli.

Posttesticular obstruction leads to increased tubule diameter, increased thickness of the tunica propria, and a decreased number of Sertoli cells and spermatids, and sometimes sloughing of the germinal epithelium.

MALE INFERTILITY TREATMENT

Because male factor is involved in approximately 50% of couples unable to conceive, it is important to evaluate and treat the male partner.

Furthermore, male infertility may also be a harbinger of a more serious underlying problem, such as cancer or endocrine problems.

Urologists, and specifically male reproductive specialists, are specially trained to evaluate and treat these issues.

MEDICAL TREATMENT

Clomiphene Citrate

It is a potent anti-estrogen, and decreases the negative feedback to the hypothalamic/pituitary axis.

This results in an increase in GnRH, and subsequently LH and FSH levels.

Testosterone is increased, as is estradiol, and in some men, sperm concentration will increase as well.

However, meta-analyses of randomized trials have failed to demonstrate an improvement in pregnancy rates with the use of clomiphene citrate in men for treatment of oligospermia.

Tamoxifen

Tamoxifen is another anti-estrogen that has a similar mechanism of action to clomiphene.

However, there is less estrogenic activity, so estradiol levels tend to be lower.

Similar to clomiphene citrate, no significant improvement in pregnancy rates have been seen in placebo-controlled trials.

Both of these drugs may be useful in men with low-normal testosterone levels.

Aromatase Inhibitors

Aromatase is the enzyme that catalyzes the conversion of testosterone to estradiol.

It is typically found in body fat; thus obese men tend to have higher circulating levels of estradiol.

Inhibition of this enzyme decreases estradiol levels, increases testosterone levels, and decreases the negative feedback from estrogen to the hypothalamic/pituitary axis.

Thus, this medication may be useful in obese men, although, no randomized trials have demonstrated an improvement in pregnancy rates.

Gonadotropins

For the treatment of hypogonadotropic hypogonadism, gonadotropin replacement using hCG, which is a LH analog, will increase the endogenous testosterone levels.

A regimen typically starts with a test dose of 1000 units of hCG given once a day subcutaneously for 5 days, followed by 500-1000 units given subcutaneously three times a week.

Testosterone levels and, if present, sperm parameters are monitored.

Once adequate testosterone levels have been achieved, FSH analog, such as hMG, is added until sperm production is noted in the semen.

The dosage is typically 75 units subcutaneously, three times a week for 3 to 6 months, until sperm appears.

Couples may then try to conceive naturally or through artificial means.

The natural conception rate for these couples is quite high, and may approach 70% in the first year.

Androgen Therapy

Administration of exogenous androgens is counterproductive, as it will increase the negative feedback to the hypothalamus and pituitary glands.

This in turn will decrease gonadotropin release, thus removing stimulation for both testosterone and sperm production. In some patients, this may lead to sterility.

Infections

Most "infections" are not really infections, but a diagnosis based on the finding of "white blood cells" in the semen.

These cells often are round cells representing immature germ cells.

However, most labs cannot differentiate the two without the use of special stains.

For patients who have true symptomatic genital infections, the semen should be cultured.

The patient should be treated with the appropriate antibiotics, typically for 4-6 weeks, and then the semen should be recultured.

This is a rare cause of male factor infertility.

Antisperm Antibodies

Patients with antisperm antibody levels greater than 1:32 may respond to immunosuppression using cyclic steroids for 3-6 months.

However, patients need to be aware of the potential side effects of steroids, including avascular necrosis of the hip, weight gain, and iatrogenic Cushing syndrome.

Retrograde Ejaculation

Imipramine or alpha-sympathomimetics, such as pseudoephedrine, may help close the bladder neck to assist in antegrade ejaculation.

However, these medicines are of limited efficacy, especially in patients with a fixed abnormality such as a bladder neck abnormality occurring after a surgical procedure.

Alternatively, sperm may be recovered from voided or catheterized postejaculatory urine to be used in assisted reproductive techniques.

The urine should be alkalinized with a solution of sodium bicarbonate for optimal recovery.

More recently, the injection of collagen to the bladder neck has allowed antegrade ejaculation in a patient who had previously undergone a V-Y plasty of the bladder neck and for whom pseudoephedrine and intrauterine insemination had failed.

Erectile Dysfunction

Treatment of erectile dysfunction should be tailored to specific patient characteristics.

It is important that underlying medical conditions are ruled out and/or treated.

Most men will respond to phosphodiesterase-5 (PDE) inhibitors (such as sildenafil); although one must be certain that the patient does not have contraindications to this treatment (for example, nitrate use).

For those who do not respond, the next step is injection therapy with vasoactive drugs, such as papaverine.

These carry a higher risk of priapism (prolonged, painful erections), so care must be taken in patient selection.

Penile implants are expensive, although satisfaction is high.

Nutritional Supplementation

Nutritional supplements typically contain carnitine, which has been shown to be present in high levels in the epididymis and may be involved in sperm motility.

Most of these compounds utilize L-carnitine, acetyl-L-carnitine or both, often in combination with other supplements, such as anti-oxidants, various vitamins and trace minerals.

Although no randomized trials have demonstrated a significant benefit in pregnancy rates, one trial showed a subset of patients with improved sperm motility.

These supplements tend not to have many side effects, although they can be somewhat expensive.

The bottom line is that these probably are not harmful, but there is no good evidence for benefit.

Lifestyle Modification

Patients should be encouraged to stop smoking cigarettes and to limit environmental exposures to harmful substances and/or conditions.

Stress-relief therapy and consultation of other appropriate psychological and social professionals may be advised.

SURGICAL TREATMENT

The three main areas of surgical treatment include varicocele, corrective surgery for obstructive azoospermia, typically either vasovasostomy (VV) or vasoepididymostomy (EV), and sperm acquisition.

Varicocele

There are three surgical approaches to varicocele repair: retroperitoneal, inguinal and subinguinal

The low inguinal/subinguinal approaches are probably the most effective with the lowest rate of recurrence and hydrocele formation.

Varicocele repair is typically an outpatient surgery performed under local, regional, or general anesthesia.

Outcomes are improved using optical magnification to preserve the spermatic artery.

Because of the spermatogenic cycle, it typically takes 3 months to see improvement following repair.

However, improvement may take 6 months in some patients.

Approximately two thirds of patients will improve, with spontaneous pregnancy rates of up to 50% when there is no female factor present.

Vasectomy Reversal

More couples are choosing to undergo vasectomy reversal, and proper technique is important.

The goal is to achieve a sperm-tight anastomosis, which requires very small sutures (typically 9-0), magnification and experience in microsurgery.

The type of anastomosis used is dependent upon the findings during surgery.

Evidence of epididymal obstruction requires anastomosis of the vas deferens to the epididymis above the point of obstruction.

Predictors of success that can be used prior to surgery to help counsel couples include time from vasectomy, experience of the microsurgeon, length of the testicular vas remnant and the age of the female partner.

The value of the presence of sperm granuloma is debated, and none of these factors are completely predictive of outcome.

Although not major surgery, vasectomy reversal is a more invasive and technically challenging procedure than a vasectomy.

It is typically performed as outpatient procedure under local, regional or general anesthesia.

The use of a surgical microscope has become the standard, although the type of repair does not affect the outcome when performed by an experienced surgeon.

In any vasectomy reversal procedure, preservation of the blood supply is essential, as well as a sperm-tight anastomosis.

The quality of the fluid helps to determine whether a vasovasostomy or vasoepididymostomy is performed.

Some of the advantages of vasectomy reversal over sperm acquisition with IVF include the ability to conceive naturally and the possibility of more than one pregnancy.

In addition, it is typically less expensive (thus more cost effective) and does not involve treatment of the female partner.

Some of the downsides to vasectomy reversal include longer time to conception (typically 6-10 months following surgery) and variable success rates based on the factors listed above.

In addition, if the procedure is unsuccessful, sperm acquisition with IVF may become necessary, and if it is successful, it may require another sterilization procedure.

Vasovasostomy

Generally, the procedure involves isolation of vasal ends, with or without delivery of the testis, taking care to preserve blood supply.

The vasal ends are brought into proximity with either vas clamps or suture, and fluid from the testicular vas is sampled.

It is necessary to utilize an operating microscope and very fine sutures due to size difference between the testicular lumen and the abdominal lumen of the vasal ends.

The outcome of vasovasostomy depends on the quality of sperm in the vas.

Vasoepididymostomy

Currently, most microsurgeons would not perform a vasovasostomy if no sperm in the vas, but rather, would go into the epididymis and perform a vasoepididymostomy.

The epididymal tubule is intussuscepted into the vasal lumen, thus creating a sperm-tight closure.

This procedure is performed in men with epididymal obstruction due to vasectomy, epididymitis, scrotal trauma, or idiopathic epididymal obstruction.

Although the success rates are not as high as with vasovasostomy, they are still successful in approximately 75% of cases.

Sperm Acquisition Techniques

When a blockage is uncorrectable, such as with congenital bilateral absence of the vas deferens (CBAVD), or if the couple elects not to correct the obstruction, sperm may be surgically retrieved from the vas deferens, epididymis or testis for use with IVF.

Most studies demonstrate that there is no difference in outcome based on site of retrieval as long as the sperm are viable.

Furthermore, in the obstructed male, most centers do not report any difference in frozen vs. freshly retrieved sperm; however, this is lab-dependent.

Microsurgical Epididymal Sperm Aspiration (MESA)

There are several indications for microsurgical epididymal sperm aspiration (MESA).

Variants of CBAVD include idiopathic epididymal obstruction, unilateral absence of the vas with contralateral absence of the seminal vesicles, or bilateral seminal vesicle agenesis.

Although some men will undergo repeat vasectomy reversal (after a previous failed vasectomy reversal) with very good success, others choose to move to IVF.

Furthermore, if the obstruction is irreparable, sperm acquisition becomes necessary.

Finally, some couples prefer not to undergo vasectomy reversal and move straight to sperm acquisition with IVF.

Some centers no longer use microsurgical epididymal sperm aspiration due to the cost and invasiveness.

However, there are still some labs that prefer motile epididymal sperm, so the procedure is still an option.

It is performed outpatient under local, regional or general anesthesia.

It does entail a scrotal incision in order to expose the epididymis, as well as an operating microscope to visualize the epididymal tubules.

Although microsurgical epididymal sperm aspiration is more invasive than other forms of sperm acquisition, it does yield high numbers (often several million) motile sperm, although typically not enough for intrauterine insemination.

Since there are usually high numbers of sperm, any extra sperm can be cryopreserved for additional cycles.

Microsurgical epididymal sperm aspiration can be performed several times, and motile sperm are retrieved in 95% of cases.

Microsurgical epididymal sperm aspiration has fallen out of favor due to the increased invasiveness, cost and the need for microsurgical expertise and instruments, including the use of an operating microscope.

Percutaneous Epididymal Sperm Aspiration (PESA)

Percutaneous epididymal sperm aspiration (PESA) is a less invasive option for obtaining epididymal sperm, with similar indications to microsurgical epididymal sperm aspiration.

It involves percutaneous aspiration of sperm from epididymis and must be utilized in conjunction with IVF.

Percutaneous epididymal sperm aspiration is typically performed under local anesthesia in the office or operating room.

The technique utilizes a 21- to 24-gauge butterfly needle, sperm wash media, and a syringe.

The epididymis is held, and multiple passes are made with needle while aspirating.

While the procedure does not require the use of magnification, there is a learning curve necessary before being able to successfully obtain motile sperm.

Percutaneous epididymal sperm aspiration has several advantages.

It is a rapid, relatively easy, non-invasive method of sperm retrieval with low cost and morbidity.

It may be performed under local anesthesia in the office and no microsurgical expertise is required.

Percutaneous epididymal sperm aspiration disadvantages include the small numbers of sperm retrieved and the possibility of diminished sperm quality due to contamination by red blood cells, thus it is typically done during an IVF treatment cycle.

Furthermore, most published reports do not have the same high success rates as other forms of sperm acquisition, although this is also lab-dependent.

Testicular Sperm Extraction/Aspiration (TESE/TESA)

Testicular sperm extraction/aspiration (TESE/TESA) has similar indications as for the microsurgical and percutaneous techniques, although it may also be used in nonobstructive azoospermia.

This technique is utilized more as labs have become more comfortable using testicular sperm.

Testicular sperm extraction/aspiration must be done in conjunction with IVF and ICSI.

Testicular sperm extraction is typically considered an open biopsy.

This approach yields significant amounts of testicular tissue, although it is more invasive than testicular sperm aspiration.

It may be most suitable for men with poor sperm production, as it allows for multiple biopsies.

Testicular sperm aspiration is a percutaneous technique.

Suction is created with the piston syringe handle.

After several passes, the needle is removed and the testis tissue is either grasped as it comes out or flushed from the tubing.

This approach will often yield enough tissue for multiple cycles and, if necessary, pathology.

Both can be performed as an outpatient under local, regional or general anesthesia, and may be performed in the office or the operating room.

Neither technique requires the use of magnification and one of two techniques may be utilized: delivery of the testis or window technique.

The testicular sperm extraction/aspiration procedure is a rapid, relatively easy, non-invasive method of sperm retrieval.

Multiple specimens can be cryopreserved for later use.

It may be performed under local anesthesia in the office and no microsurgical expertise required.

Disadvantage of testicular sperm extraction/aspiration is that the lab must be familiar/comfortable working with testicular sperm.

Testicular sperm aspiration is not always successful, and may need to be converted to an open extraction procedure.

Microscopic Testicular Sperm Extraction (Micro-TESE)

Microscopic testicular sperm extraction (also called micro-TESE) is based on the finding that tubules that contain sperm appear larger under an operating microscope than those that do not.

Therefore, it is possible to identify these tubules and remove them without removing large pieces of testicular tissue.

Because of the localized nature of sperm production in nonobstructive azoospermia, the other forms of sperm acquisition, for example, MESA and PESA are not utilized in these patients.

ASSISTED REPRODUCTION TECHNIQUES

Artificial Insemination

Artificial insemination (AI) involves the placement of sperm directly into the cervix (intracervical insemination [ICI]) or the uterus (intrauterine insemination [IUI]).

AI is most useful for couples in whom who have very low sperm density or motility, or those who have unexplained infertility.

IUI allows the sperm to be placed past the inhospitable cervical mucus and increases the chance of natural fertilization.

This results in a 4% pregnancy rate if used alone and a pregnancy rate of 8-17% if combined with superovulation.

Both processes require semen processing.

Patients in whom IUI has failed 3-6 times should consider proceeding to IVF.

In Vitro Fertilization (IVF)

IVF involves fertilization of the egg outside the body and reimplantation of the fertilized embryo into the woman's uterus.

Indications for IVF include previous failures with IUI and known conditions of the male or female precluding the use of less-demanding techniques.

IVF generally requires a minimum of 50,000-500,000 motile sperm.

Harvesting eggs initially involves down-regulating the woman's pituitary with a GnRH agonist and then performing ovarian hyperstimulation.

Follicular development is monitored by ultrasonographic examination and by checking serum levels of estrogen and progesterone.

When the follicles are appropriately enlarged, a transvaginal follicular aspiration is performed.

A mean of 12 eggs are typically retrieved per cycle, and they are immediately placed in an agar of fallopian-tube medium.

After an incubation period of 3-6 hours, the sperm are added to the medium using approximately 100,000 sperm per oocyte.

After 48 hours, the embryos have usually reached the 3- to 8-cell stage.

Two to 4 embryos are usually implanted in the uterus, while the remaining embryos are frozen for future use.

Pregnancy rates are 10-45%.

Overall, IVF is a safe and useful procedure.

Risks include multiple pregnancies and hyperstimulation syndrome.

Gamete/Zygote Intrafallopian Transfer (GIFT/ZIFT)

These procedures allow the placement of semen (GIFT) or a fertilized zygote (ZIFT) directly into the fallopian tube by laparoscopy.

Success rates have been estimated to be 25-30% using these techniques.

Unfortunately, these procedures require general anesthesia and have associated risks.

Fertilization and implantation are not guaranteed, and these procedures cannot be performed in patients with fallopian tube obstruction.

GIFT and ZIFT are rarely used as a therapeutic option.

Intracytoplasmic Sperm Injection (ICSI)

ICSI involves the direct injection of a sperm into an egg under microscopy.

It is indicated in patients who have failed more conservative therapies or those with severe abnormalities including patients with sperm extracted directly from the epididymis or testicle.

Oocytes are processed with hyaluronidase to remove the cumulus mass and corona radiata.

A micropipette is used to hold the egg while a second micropipette injects the sperm.

The oocyte is positioned with the polar body at the 6-o'clock or 12-o'clock position, and the sperm is injected at the 3-o'clock position to minimize the risk of chromosomal damage in the egg.

After incubation for 48 hours, the embryo is implanted in the woman.

A 59% fertilization rate and a 35% pregnancy rate with the use of ICSI was reported.

Fresh sperm and cryopreserved sperm appear to have similar success rates.

In female partners of men with infertility who are undergoing ICSI, diminished ovarian reserve may adversely affect the success of TESE.

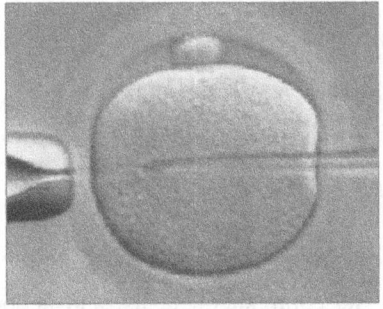

Intracytoplasmic Sperm Injection (ICSI)

MALE FERTILITY PRESERVATION

Cancer is not common in men of reproductive age; however, it is an important cause of morbidity, particularly male infertility.

As more of these cancers are cured, these men live longer and thus experience issues with infertility.

Therefore, preservation of their reproductive function is an important part of the treatment plan in these men.

Induction of infertility, as well as the degree of recovery, is due to multiple factors, including the type of treatment (chemotherapy, radiation, or surgery), the duration of treatment and the degree of injury, as well as underlying issues.

Most men who recover do so within the first 2-3 years, although it may take as long as 10 years to overcome all of these effects.

Testicular Cancer

Testicular cancer is the most common solid tumor in men of reproductive age.

Because of the advances in treatment, there is a very high cure rate (typically over 90%), so these men are now surviving and desiring fertility.

However, due to several factors, including cryptorchidism, systemic disease, disease in the contralateral testis, and endocrine abnormalities due to some of the tumor markers produced, nearly half of these men have a reduction in their baseline fertility prior to treatment.

Effects of Therapy

Radical orchiectomy, the first step in treatment, removes half of the testicular tissue.

Fortunately, most men remain fertile if no other therapy is required.

In the case of bilateral tumors or in men who have already lost a testis, partial orchiectomy is feasible if the tumor is small, localized, and the patient is willing to undergo rigorous surveillance.

Adjuvant treatment after orchiectomy, such as radiation, chemotherapy, or retroperitoneal lymph node dissection (RPLND), may further damage fertility in these men.

The nerves that control ejaculation (the sympathetic trunk) run along the aorta and can be damaged by surgery to that area.

In the case of testis cancer, this is where the lymph nodes that drain the testes lie, and the sympathetic trunk must be carefully dissected away from the lymph nodes in order to preserve ejaculatory function.

Because ejaculation is mediated by the sympathetic nervous system, injury to the sympathetic trunk can result in ejaculatory dysfunction, including anejaculation (no semen coming out) or retrograde ejaculation.

The risk of this is related to the surgical technique, as well as the type of retroperitoneal lymph node dissection performed.

The risk of ejaculatory dysfunction is nearly 100% in men undergoing this procedure after chemotherapy due to the desmoplastic response of the tumor, thus obliterating the nerves.

If a modified template (which typically spares one side of the nerves) is used for retroperitoneal lymph node dissection (without chemotherapy), the risk is still 10 to 20%.

However, if a bilateral nerve-sparing retroperitoneal lymph node dissection is performed by a surgeon skilled in this technique, the risk of ejaculatory dysfunction is less than 5%.

Preventive Measures

Preventive measures for men undergoing such procedures include banking sperm prior to any therapy and limiting radiation exposure and shielding testes during treatments.

If possible, chemotherapeutic agents with less effect on germinal epithelium should be utilized.

Patients requiring retroperitoneal surgery should be referred to experts in this area (not generalists).

Post-treatment Fertility Options

After treatment, fertility options are dependent upon whether or not there is sperm present in the ejaculate, the quality of the semen, and whether or not sperm was cryopreserved prior to treatment.

Various techniques can be performed in order to obtain sperm following testicular cancer treatment.

If the patient has retrograde ejaculation, alpha-agonists, such as pseudoephedrine, or sympathomimetics, such as imipramine, may induce antegrade ejaculation.

If retrograde ejaculation is still present, the urine may be alkalinized in order to protect the sperm and post-ejaculate urine may be collected.

If no ejaculate is present, then techniques including vibratory stimulation, electroejaculation (EEJ), vasal/epididymal/seminal vesicle aspiration and testicular sperm extraction (TESE/TESA) may be utilized.

Recommendations

All cancer patients should be directed to cryopreserve sperm prior to starting any type of cancer treatment.

The number of ejaculates cryopreserved should be dependent upon the expected post-thaw yield.

Patients should also be instructed to refrain from conception for at least 6 to 12 months following radiation or chemotherapy.

In addition, patients should be counseled as to the length of time necessary for recovery of spermatogenesis.

Patients should be counseled about banking sperm; if they are able to provide ejaculated sample, they should do so; if unable, they should be referred for potential sperm retrieval.

Efforts should be made to minimize surgical/medical morbidity; do not assume that shielding/dose reduction will prevent problems; also, surgical technique matters.

Finally, microsurgery and assisted reproductive technology can overcome even severe abnormalities.

REFERENCES

– Abdel-Meguid TA, Al-Sayyad A, Tayib A, et al. Does varicocele repair improve male infertility? An evidence-based perspective from a randomized, controlled trial. Eur Urol. 2011; 59: 455-61.

– Agarwal A, Prabakaran SA, Said TM. Prevention of Oxidative Stress Injury to Sperm. Journal of Andrology. 2005; 26: 654-60.

– Al Bakri A, Lo K, Grober E, et al. Time for improvement in semen parameters after varicocelectomy. J Urol. 2012; 187: 227-31.

– Anger JT, Goldstein M. Intravasal "toothpaste" in men with obstructive azoospermia is derived from vasal epithelium, not sperm. J Urol. 2004; 172: 634-6.

– Baccetti BM, Bruni E, Capitani S, et al. Studies on varicocele III: ultrastructural sperm evaluation and 18, X and Y aneuploidies. J Androl. 2006; 27: 94-101.

– Berookhim BM, Mulhall JP. Outcomes of operative sperm retrieval strategies for fertility preservation among males scheduled to undergo cancer treatment. Fertil Steril. 2014; 101: 805-11.

– Bhasin S, Mallidis C, Ma K. The genetic basis of infertility in men. Baillieres Best Pract Res Clin Endocrinol Metab. 2000; 14: 363-388.

– Bouloux P, Warne DW, Loumaye E; FSH Study Group in Men's Infertility. Efficacy and safety of recombinant human follicle-stimulating hormone in men with isolated hypogonadotropic hypogonadism. Fertil Steril. 2002; 77: 270-3.

– Brackett NL, Lynne CM, Aballa TC, et al. Sperm motility from the vas deferens of spinal cord injured men is higher than from the ejaculate. J Urol. 2000; 164: 712-5.

– Brugh VM, Lipshultz LI. Male factor infertility. Medical Clinics of North America. 2004; 88(2): 367-85.

– Carmignani L, Gadda F, Mancini M, et al. Detection of testicular ultrasonographic lesions in severe male infertility. J Urol. 2004; 172: 1045-7.

References

- Cavallini G. Male idiopathic oligoasthenoteratozoospermia. Asian Journal of Andrology. 2006; 8: 143-57.

- Chung KW. Gross Anatomy. 4th ed. Philadelphia: Lippincott Williams & Wilkins; 2000.

- Cooper TG, Noonan E, von Eckardstein S, et al. World Health Organization reference values for human semen characteristics. Hum Reprod Update. 2010; 16: 231-45.

- Cooper TG, Noonan E, Von Eckardstein S, et al. World Health Organization reference values for human semen characteristics. Human Reproduction Update. 2009; 16: 231-45.

- Costabile RA, Spevak M. Characterization of patients presenting with male factor infertility in an equal access, no cost medical system. Urology. 2001; 58: 1021-4.

- Drake RL, Vogl AW, Mitchell AWM. Gray's Anatomy for Student's. 2nd ed. Philadelphia: Churchill Livingstone Elsevier; 2010.

- Eisenberg ML, Betts P, Herder D, et al. Increased risk of cancer among azoospermic men. Fertil Steril. 2013; 100: 681-5.

- Fenig DM, Kattan MW, Mills JN, et al. Nomogram to preoperatively predict the probability of requiring epididymovasostomy during vasectomy reversal. J Urol. 2012; 187: 215-8.

- Fretz PC, Sandlow JI: Varicocele-Current concepts in pathophysiology, diagnosis and treatment. In Lipshultz LI (ed.): Urologic Clinics of North America. Philadelphia: WB Saunders; 2002.

- Gaur DS, Talekar M, Pathak VP. Effect of cigarette smoking on semen quality of infertile men. Singapore Medical Journal. 2007; 48: 119-23.

- Gillen- water JY, Grayhack JT, Howards SS, et al, editors. Adult and pediatric urology. 4th ed. London: Lippincott. Williams & Wilkins; 2002.

References

− Gillen-water JY, Grayhack JT, Howards SS, et al. Adult and pediatric urology. 4th ed. London: Lippincott. Williams & Wilkins; 2002.

− Giwercman A, Petersen PM. Cancer and male infertility. Baillieres Best Pract Res Clin Endocrinol Metab. 2000; 14: 453-471.

− Hauser R, Yogev L, Amit A, et al. Severe hypospermatogenesis in cases of nonobstructive azoospermia: should we use fresh or frozen testicular spermatozoa? J Androl. 2005; 26: 772-8.

− Hauser R, Yogev L, Paz G, et al. Comparison of efficacy of two techniques for testicular sperm retrieval in nonobstructive azoospermia: multifocal testicular sperm extraction versus multifocal testicular sperm aspiration. J Androl. 2006; 27: 28-33.

− Hirsh A. Male subfertility. BMJ. 2003; 327: 669-72.

− Hsiao W, Sultan R, Lee R, Goldstein M. Increased follicle-stimulating hormone is associated with higher assisted reproduction use after vasectomy reversal. J Urol. 2011; 185: 2266-71.

− Hwang K, Walters RC, Lipshultz LI. Contemporary concepts in the evaluation and management of male infertility. Nature Reviews Urology. 2011; 8: 86-94.

− Jacobsen KD, Theodorsen L, Fossa SD. Spermatogenesis after unilateral orchiectomy for testicular cancer in patients following surveillance policy. J Urol. 2001; 165: 93-6.

− Katz VL, Lentz GM, Lobo RA, et al. Comprehensive Gynecology. 5th ed. Philadelphia: Mosby Elsevier; 2007.

− Keel BA. Within- and between-subject variation in semen parameters in infertile men and normal semen donors. Fertil Steril. 2006; 85: 128-34.

− Klemetti R, Gissler M, Sevon T, et al. Children born after assisted fertilization have an increased rate of major congenital anomalies. Fertil Steril. 2005; 84: 1300-7.

− Leibovitch I, Mor Y. The Vicious Cycling: Bicycling Related Urogenital Disorders. European Urology. 2005; 47: 277-86.

References

— Lipshultz LI, Rumohr JA, Bennett RC. Techniques for Vasectomy Reversal. In Sandlow JI and Nagler HN (eds.): Urologic Clinics of North America. Philadelphia: WB Saunders; 2009.

— Lombardo F, Sansone A, Romanelli F, et al. The role of antioxidant therapy in the treatment of male infertility: An overview. Asian Journal of Andrology. 2011; 13: 690-7.

— Loukas M, Colburn GL, Abrahams P, et al. Gray's Anatomy Review. Philadelphia: Churchill Livingstone Elsevier; 2010.

— Male Infertility Best Practice Policy Committee of the American Urological Association; Practice Committee of the American Society for Reproductive Medicine. Report on optimal evaluation of the infertile male. Fertil Steril. 2006; 86: S202-9.

— McCallum TJ, Milunsky JM, Cunningham DL, et al. Fertility in men with cystic fibrosis: an update on current surgical practices and outcomes. Chest. 2000; 118: 1059-62.

— Mills JN, Meacham RB. Nonsurgical Treatment of male infertility. In Lipshultz L, Howards S, and Niederberger C (eds). Infertility in the Male, 4th ed. Cambridge: Cambridge University Press; 2009.

— Neill J. Knobil and Neill's Physiology of Reproduction. 3rd ed. St. Louis, MO: Elsevier; 2006.

— Olson CK, Keppler KM, Romitti PA, et al. In vitro fertilization is associated with an increase in major birth defects. Fertil Steril. 2005; 84: 1308-15.

— Omurtag K, Cooper A, Bullock A, et al. Sperm recovery and IVF after testicular sperm extraction (TESE): effect of male diagnosis and use of off-site surgical centers on sperm recovery and IVF. PLoS One. 2013; 8: e69838.

— Ovalle WK, Nahirney PC. Netter's Eseential Histology. Philadelphia: Sauders Elsevier; 2007.

– Pasqualotto FF, Sobreiro BP, Hallak J, et al. Induction of spermatogenesis in azoospermic men after varicocelectomy repair: an update. Fertil Steril. 2006; 85: 635-9.

– Practice Committee of the American Society for Reproductive Medicine. Report on management of obstructive azoospermia. Fertil Steril. 2006; 86: S259-63.

– Purohit RS, Wu DS, Shinohara K, et al. A prospective comparison of 3 diagnostic methods to evaluate ejaculatory duct obstruction. J Urol. 2004; 171: 232-5.

– Raman JD, Nobert CF, Goldstein M. Increased incidence of testicular cancer in men presenting with infertility and abnormal semen analysis. J Urol. 2005; 174: 1819-22.

– Sadler T.W. Langman's Medical Embryology. 11th ed. Baltimore, Maryland: Lippincott Williams & Wilkins; 2010.

– Safarinejad MR, Safarinejad S, Shafiei N, et al. Effects of the reduced form of coenzyme q(10) (ubiquinol) on semen parameters in men with idiopathic infertility: a double-blind, placebo controlled, randomized study. J Urol. 2012; 188: 526-31.

– Salzhauer EW, Sokol A, Glassberg KI. Paternity after adolescent varicocele repair. Pediatrics. 2004; 114: 1631-3.

– Schatte EC, Orejuela FJ, Lipshultz LI, et al. Treatment of infertility due to anejaculation in the male with electroejaculation and intracytoplasmic sperm injection. J Urol. 2000; 163: 1717-20.

– Spitz A, Kim ED, Lipshultz LI. Contemporary approach to the male infertility evaluation. Obstet Gynecol Clin North Am. 2000; 27: 487-516, v.

– Standring S. Gray's Anatomy. 40th ed. Edinburgh: Elsevier Churchill Livingstone; 2008.

– Teerds KJ, de Rooij DG, Keijer J. Functional relationship between obesity and male reproduction: from humans to animal models. Human Reproduction Update. 2011; 17: 667-83.

References

– Traber MG, Stevens JF. Vitamins C and E: Beneficial effects from a mechanistic perspective. Free Radical Biology and Medicine. 2011; 51: 1000-13.

– Vicdan A, Vicdan K, Günalp S, et al. Genetic aspects of human male infertility: the frequency of chromosomal abnormalities and Y chromosome microdeletions in severe male factor infertility. Eur J Obstet Gynecol Reprod Biol. 2004; 117: 49-54.

– Wald M, Ross LS, Prins GS, et al. Analysis of outcomes of cryopreserved surgically retrieved sperm for IVF/ICSI. J Androl. 2006; 27: 60-5.

– Wein AJ, ed. Campbell-Walsh Urology. 9th ed. Philadelphia, Pa: Saunders Elsevier; 2007.

– Wein AJ. Campbell-Walsh Urology. 9th ed. Philadelphia: Saunders Elsevier; 2007.

– Whitten SJ, Nangia AK, Kolettis PN. Select patients with hypogonadotropic hypogonadism may respond to treatment with clomiphene citrate. Fertil Steril. 2006; 86: 1664-8.

– World Health Organization. WHO Laboratory Manual for the Examination of Human Semen and Sperm Cervical Mucus Interaction. 4th ed. Cambridge, United Kingdom: Cambridge Unviersity Press; 1999.

– Zahalsky MP, Berman AJ, Nagler HM. Evaluating the risk of epididymal injury during hydrocelectomy and spermatocelectomy. J Urol. 2004; 171: 2291-2.

www.ingramcontent.com/pod-product-compliance
Lightning Source LLC
Chambersburg PA
CBHW071755170526
45167CB00003B/1040

Male factors are often the cause of a couple's failure to conceive therefore, it is important to evaluate and treat the male partner. A male factor may be due to abnormalities of hormonal control, testicular function, or sperm transport or delivery.

Evaluation of infertile men is essential to identify both correctable and uncorrectable conditions.

A thorough medical and reproductive history and physical examination are integral parts of the workup.

The semen analysis provides the basis for identifying the cause of male infertility, as well as planning additional testing and treatment.

Treatment options are based on the underlying etiology and range from optimizing semen production and transportation with medical therapy or surgical procedures to complex assisted reproduction techniques.

I hope this book will enhance your knowledge of male infertility and you will be able to apply this information to your practice.

Prof. Dr. Akmal Nabil Ahmad El-Mazny, MD, FICS
Professor of Obstetrics and Gynecology
Consultant of Reproductive and Endoscopic Surgery
Faculty of Medicine, Cairo University, Egypt